I CARE FOR ME FIRST

I CARE FOR ME FIRST

My Rx to Self-Care

SYRENTHIA COLINO

DEDICATION

This book is dedicated to all the caregivers who continuously show up, putting themselves second. May this book be a tool in your toolkit and remind you that you too should be first.

CONTENTS

INTRODUCTION

From 11.0% to 41.1%.
Those percentages represent the average share of adults who reported anxiety disorder symptoms and depressive disorder according to the NHIS Early Release Program and the U.S. Census Bureau Household Pulse Survey.

What time frame was this, you might be asking? The 11% was from January 2019 to June 2019, while the 41.1% was from January 2021. So there was an almost 4x jump of people, and as you guess, the pandemic and Covid-19 were smack at the center of why this was the case.

While many people were struggling with their mental health, the conversation about self-care also grew and rose to levels never seen before. You could not turn on the television and not see episode after episode of these statistics materializing in real life. Many of those first responders were at the forefront of the news. We honored many of them for courageously standing on the frontlines and helping others navigate the pandemic despite the ramifications it could have on their health.

Many in the profession are now receiving their capes and being called heroes while doing this work all along. But, what was new to many was not new to those who are caregivers. For many years, caregivers worldwide have swept under the rug their health, placing it second or even last, so that those they care for would be put first. While a new pandemic brought to light the need for mental health and self-care, this epidemic of not taking care of yourself first or equally giving yourself care was part of the same ol' same ol', which struck my core.

As you will learn more in-depth in the book, I'm a parent who has experienced severe and adverse reactions and psychological trauma because of my ignorance of understanding the signs of burnout and emotional fatigue. You're probably not as familiar with the term "emotional fatigue" as with physical exhaustion, but this is more real than you can imagine. Fatigue is often only looked at from a physical sense. Still, the emotional weight of fatigue could equally be just as heavy, if not heavier, because many people never truly understand it because it's not always seen. It took others calling out my burnout for me even to realize that I was experiencing it myself. This goes to show the danger of it. Like many other diseases labeled as silent killers, ignoring your self-care can also produce the same unfortunate consequences to our well-being.

For this reason, I decided that a book like this was needed. A book that would advocate for special needs parents and caregivers' self-care. First responders who are also like caregivers on a broader scope too could benefit from what this book highlights. For far too long, our duty has been tied to the service of others only, even if it was to the detriment of our very own well-being.

No longer can we look at self-care as something done only after something happens, and not enough is done to speak of it as preventive health care. Many people are burning out in their roles as caregivers. People are either quitting the profession or on the brink of mental, emotional, spiritual, or physical breakdown that they may not be able to bounce back from. It's said that there are two great times for change, 20 years ago and right now. The people this book is written for don't have another 20 years going with the flow as they are right now; they simply won't make it.

When you read this book, you won't just listen to my account of when and how self-care came to my awareness, but you'll be able to identify the similarities of how it may show up for you. For example, an account of burnout through someone else's eyes might turn the light on for you and help you realize that you, too, are in the middle of your self-care struggle. Also, you'll find thought-provoking questions that will help you no longer have a blind spot when it comes to your own care. Once you have that new awareness of where you are in your self-care journey, then and only then are you ready to appreciate its value and dive into a personalized plan of what it looks like for you. My journey simply is a shadow or reflection of what could be and should be as a caregiver, an invitation, if you will, to the life you could have and should have. You'll finally feel seen, felt, and heard of the struggles you've had of putting your care second or, even worse, last, and ready to no longer be your reality.

CHAPTER 1

SELF-CARE 911

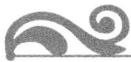

As a mother of two children, one on the autism spectrum, I was challenged to practice self-care. My day consisted of medical billing and caring for a typical and non-typical kid; while having 3 hours of sleep a night. Most people complain about the sleepless nights; there were no such complaints from me. Instead, I was grateful that I was able to get some sleep. I became a caregiver at the age of 20, raising a son who was newly diagnosed with autism in the late 90s. I had no clue what to do, and there was little local support during this time. While the local support was not available, I don't know where I would have been without the wonderful and amazing grandmother I had, who supported me from a distance; what most people do not know is that when you are caregiving for a loved one, you must take some alone time whether it is 30 minutes or an hour. You need that time to step away to prevent burnout from your day-to-day routine. This is something that caregivers may or may not know but rarely put into practice or feel like they have the privilege to put into practice.

When the kids turned 18 and 20, I saw it as my opportunity to get out of the house and go into the working world. Before that, I was working from home full-time. In 2007, I decided to take a job at one of the major insurance corporations. I felt the need to socialize with other adults in the workforce. Now, this was an eye-opener about life for me. I experience everything possible while working this 9 am-5 pm job. I learned that I had so many things going on with me but covered up for years since I did not take the time to deal with my emotions. I did not have the time for myself. I was too busy raising autism, supporting my kids and household along with other family members; I did not know how to care for the most important person, which was me. After working in the office setting for a year, everything was going great, and the kids needed me less, mainly my son. I went from a Young Mother raising two kids on my own to a woman who had all these emotions but had no idea how to care for them or what to do with them. I realize that I started having too much available time and did not know how to fill this time with things to do. You've probably heard the saying that idle time is the devil's playground, right? Well, here I was with idle time, and it felt like my emotions were running wild, having me feel all over the place.

Fast to 3 years later, being away from home and getting settled working in an office, you would think that my emotions and handling of things would have gotten better, but actually, the opposite occurred.

Summer 2010 was when the breaking point started. After a long week of being emotional at the office, shedding tears without any reason, not being able to complete any of my tasks, and pacing up and down the hallway, Edna, the office manager, called me in her office since mine was right next to hers and said, "*Are you ok Syrenthia, is there anything I can assist you with? I notice that you're having a challenging day, actually a week, which is unlike you.*" My response was that I just needed a little air, so I took a walk outside since this had been going on for months, being so emotional, having sweating hands, having palpitations, and feeling overwhelmed overall. Edna asks, "Where are your family or friends that can give you the support you need when you're having such a day?" My answer to her was my Granny, and she is not local, and I would be sure to give her a call when I get to the house. She was the full support I needed, even if she was long-distance. Granny was the spiritual support I needed to give me that balance, but that only lasted for a day or two, and I'll be right back in the same state I was in. So after answering Edna, I headed outside for that fresh air. I gave her that I'm ok smile, and I walked down the hallway toward the elevator, thinking about how I've become so numb in allowing myself to not be emotional in front of anyone. Once I got outside, I could talk myself out of having a panic attack. This was something that I started having two years into working at ABC, but I overlooked it as I often did when it came to ME. I noticed all the emotional breakdown was coming on every time I walked through the door of that building, but I ignored the signs since I was just happy to be around other adults, which I hadn't been in years.

After the workday ended, I headed to the house, where I felt relieved when I walked through my door. It was as if nothing had happened earlier that day. My house was my safety zone; it's where I knew what was going to happen and how to manage the different energies I lived with. Leaving the house and working in the office presented me with a new challenge, handling so many people with different energies that I had to learn to manage and take on. This experience woke me up to how to deal with others and what not to take on.

Now at home, as I got settled, I decided to give my granny a call. This call was particularly tough because I had just faced one of the worst days, and it exposed how emotionally unstable I was. This shook me more than I thought, as I felt that after 20 years of raising autism that this was something I could easily manage, but that was not the case. Granny and connection was very strong; it was a connection unlike no other. She was the one who helped me get through the challenging times of raising Autism back in 1990, especially since the support from other places was nowhere to be found. Granny's support was straightforward. She held no punches and would not sugarcoat anything for me. She said, "look, baby pull yourself together and work on YOU. Stop giving yourself to others and having nothing left for you. Work more on your Spiritual well-being and set boundaries." So I see why she encouraged me to work outside of the house. She saw it as an opportunity for me to work on ME after so many years of caring for two individuals and not doing anything for myself.

This conversation with granny was a little different from the usual ones. It didn't center around the kids, not even Stephen, who she loved dearly. We spoke about various things, but I also learned that she was hospital-bound. Unfortunately, she didn't share this with me until the end of the conversation. That is when I learned she was ill, which cut our conversation short that day.

FALL 2010

A month after speaking with granny and knowing she wasn't in her best health, I had another panic attack at work, and the only co-worker I was talkative with suggested that I take a walk and she would come along with me until I felt calm. Aisha said, "Hey Syrenthia, you should maybe take a week off and go and see your granny." This was the first time I felt as if someone besides my granny was in my corner looking out for me. So I took Aisha's advice and requested a week off to go and visit my granny.

I left LA the next day to see my granny in the hospital. When I walked into the hospital room, the feeling was plain magical. There are no words I could write that would do our connection justice, but it was so strong that even if we didn't speak verbally, our eyes had their own language.

As you could imagine seeing her in the hospital, all I wanted to do was make it all about her, but she would have none of that. She never liked me fussing over her because she reinforced that idea of me caring for someone else and not caring for me first. During the week I visited Granny, it was the most peaceful week I've had in such a long time. There were no panic attacks, stress, or feelings of depression, just pure joy. Before my flight back to LA, I stopped to see her, and she said to me, "Baby, just love on you a little more since you looked so tired when you got here. Make sure you read the Psalm scriptures I've given you throughout the years, and no matter what anybody tells you, talk to your GOD, your higher power; this will always keep you grounded and connected spiritually. Oh! And remember no one can fix you but you." This was something she would always tell me before the end of every phone call. I now know exactly what she was talking about. It took me going through such a painful experience to learn I can't continue fixing others and leaving my care in the hands of others.

THE CALL

Seven days after being back in LA, I received a phone call that left me uneasy. It was a call from my Granny, and that call would be the last of the many phone calls I received from her. It was on that very day she transitioned. So many thoughts ran through my head. Suddenly, my most vital connection that brought me peace and calm was no longer here. I could feel the panic attack coming. What was I to do with the sweaty palms, my heart racing like I was at a Nascar racetrack? My safety shield was no longer here to talk me through the complexities of this world. Little did I know that she had been preparing me for this day for so long. I thought she supported me by raising my son on the spectrum, but she was preparing me to take better care of myself.

Monday came around, and it was time to leave my safety net, aka my home, and go off to the office. The first 4 hours were not bad at all. I was able to keep it together. In the 5th hour, however, I can't say the same happened. I received a phone call from a client, and something in the call triggered me into a crying spell. Aisha, my co-worker, heard my phone call and got the attention of the office manager to come to see what was going on. She was there in a blink of an eye. For some reason, I think she was just keeping a strong eye on me since most of the co-workers were whispering among themselves about the emotional episode I had a couple of months ago. Edna came into the office and asked me to put the client on hold, and she took over the call. After the call, she said, "you go and take a couple of days off," and suggested I talk to someone about how I was feeling. My emotion took over me from years of being bottled up and not expressing myself or dealing with the situation. After being off for two days and doing nothing but getting in and out of bed, I decided to call and schedule an appointment to see a therapist. That is where My RX for Self-Care 911 began.

Before moving on to the next chapter, I've included questions about Self-Care (911) questions. I often ask these questions when talking with other caregivers about their self-care. It's an opportunity for you to do some self-reflection and bring awareness to your level of self-care. Awareness is one of the first steps toward being able to care for yourself first.

SELF-CARE (911) QUESTIONS

1. What are some ways that you would define a caregiver?
2. How are you currently caring for yourself to prevent or experience burnout?
3. Where would you say that you are in your spiritual journey?
4. How can you show more gratitude and be more self-aware to shape your life?
5. What are some signs that would let you know someone is emotionally depleted?

SELF-CARE CHRONICLES

I met Syrenthia on June 13, 2018. It was a beautiful morning, and we sat down for a cup of tea. She was looking for a new Social Media Manager, and I was looking for a unique opportunity. We had an instant connection. Syrenthia has been a refreshing inspiration in many areas of my life.

Sometimes we text or email each other simultaneously, saying the same thing or answering the other person's question before the question has even been asked. She is so in tune with herself and the needs of other people. We have shared many fun times when we laugh until our stomachs hurt, and our cheeks are sore. She has taught me to have better boundaries with everyone around me.

She taught me to embrace self-care no matter the day and not feel guilty for needing time to myself no matter the day. In addition, she has been supportive through relationship and friendship troubles while instilling a sense of integrity and awareness.

The friendship we have developed over the years is so special to me. Every time we talk, she shares pieces of wisdom without giving advice; she shares similar stories relatable to what I may be experiencing, and we can laugh about it. One of the essential things she has taught me is that laughter is truly the best medicine.

Thank you, Syrenthia, for being a fantastic friend and bringing out the best in me and so many other people. The world is a better place because you are in it and the incredible gift you give just by being you.

JENNIFER MCDOUGALL
Lifestyle Blogger + Social Media Manager

CHAPTER 2

PRACTICING SELF-CARE

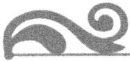

*"When you care about something that
nourishes your soul and brings joy to your
life, make room for it in your life"*
—Jean Shinoda Bolen

It was a warm day and my first appointment with Dr. Stephen Moore. I arrived at his office at 8:15 am for my 8:30 am appointment. Since it was my first experience with a therapist, I wanted to catch a glimpse of his demeanor and personality. When Dr. Moore pulled up in the parking lot, he drove a black Acura without tinted windows.

At first sight, I was taken back. His hair was unkempt and all over the place. He was wearing a pair of True Religion blue jeans and UGG boots. As I stepped out of the car, I held back my laughter because I could not believe that this was the person who was going to help me. He looked like he needed help! I was skeptical but little did I know he would lead me on a journey of self-care, self-healing, and self-love. Finally, we headed upstairs into his office. As I walked in, I smelt amazing essential oils as I walked in and heard calming sounds playing through the speakers. His office gave off a feeling of peace, tranquility, and stillness.

As soon as we began the introductions, I looked out the window to the beautiful view below, and tears streamed down my face. Dr. Moore reassured me that everything would be alright, and I gave him a little smile to let him know that I was ok. Forty minutes into the session, I am gazing out the window with a blank stare. I glanced over at Dr. Moore, and I noticed that he was sitting in a yoga pose in the corner of his office! I could not believe how peaceful he was. I rolled my eyes toward the window and thought, "How does one get to such a peaceful place?"

I was a little upset about how calm and relaxed he was while I had so many emotions running through my body. As we neared the end of my visit, Dr. Moore asked me if there was anything that I would like to discuss. I shook my head "no" and let him know that I was good while so many thoughts ran through my head. We scheduled our appointment for the following Saturday. Dr. Moore reminded me about his late appointment change policies as I rushed to leave the office. I left the office with a smirk and thought, "Maybe I can get through these sessions."

The following Saturday, walking into my appointment, Dr. Moore was sitting there in his yoga pose, meditating, and waiting for me. As I sat down quietly in his calm office, waiting for him to finish his meditating session, he opened one eye, smiled, and nodded to acknowledge my presence.

As soon as he acknowledged I was there, tears rolled down my face. The thought of sharing how I felt was so terrifying to me. After experiencing so many days of feeling overwhelmed, having panic attacks, and crying for no reason, I felt a little at ease by being around him, but it would be a process for that ease to increase to the level I needed it to be. Ten minutes into our session, as I was dazing out of the window into a beautiful view, Dr. Moore asked me to tell him about myself. During the entire week, I analyzed what I would talk about during our visit and the things that were off-limits for me. I gave the list to Dr. Moore, and he looked at me with a blank face as if I was joking. In my heart, I wanted to share everything with him, but my mind was in control, and I was unprepared to speak about triggering topics. Being vulnerable was not something that I often did. It took three years of therapy with Dr. Moore to be able to do this. Finally, for some reason, I was able to communicate with him and disconnect simultaneously, but he was beyond patient with me. He was never in a rush during our visits, as most clinical professionals usually are when seeing a challenging patient.

"Well, You know my name, Syrenthia. I have two kids. One son on the Autism Spectrum and a typical daughter."

"Tell me more about yourself." "What do you do in your downtime?"

I couldn't respond to the questions at once, so I shut down and refused to speak for the rest of our appointment. I bluntly cut him off and decided that I was done with this conversation. Rather than feeling offended, Dr. Moore went back into his yoga pose and began meditating.

As time passed, I learned that he did this regularly during our sessions. I did not mind. As I watched the clock on the wall, I mentioned that our visit was up. He asked if I would like to make another appointment with him, and I said yes. I decided that I wanted to attend therapy every Saturday morning from that point on. While walking out of the door that day, I turned around, jokingly, and said, "Hey, Dr. Moore! I will do this in my downtime, come down and not talk to you!"

After five months of small talk, not speaking, and Dr. Moore meditating, I finally broke down and opened up to him. Our first discussion was about my Granny and how I was shaped to be an amazing mother due to her support from a distance. She was a vessel of my higher power from God, and I'm so grateful that he loves me so much to have blessed me with that needed support. We laughed together about her method of raising Autism from a distance, and she was constantly on me about taking care of myself.

Our conversation led to the question I had been asked 23 visits ago, "What do you do in your downtime?" I did not have much of an answer. Upon ending our visit, Dr. Moore gave me the task, or homework, or doing something for myself as often as possible.

Leading up to 6 months of sessions with Dr. Moore, he asked me on the 24th visit about what I did for myself when I first woke up in the mornings besides the everyday things.

"Well, after doing my basic morning routine, I chat with my higher power GOD. I do this before I exchange any energy outside of me."

"You finally started doing your homework," he said.

I would receive a weekly homework task to decrease my stress levels. Then, he would educate me on caring for ME first. After that, I made a point of doing one or two things for myself monthly.

Whether it was dining out alone or taking walks around my neighborhood at any point in the day, I went from being utterly isolated to completely socializing a little. Leaving the house alone to spend a little time with myself became regular.

Caring for me became so easy to do and part of my daily routine. In the summer of 2011, I started attending cardio "Drenched" classes three times a week and boxing classes once a week. Mr. Blanks and the Drenched family fitness classes were instrumental during the start of my fitness journey. Mr. Blanks was the most patient person ever when training me. He knew that I was raising autism and made it a point to work his private training around my schedule. There were days that I would go home sore and try to make excuses not to go back, but he did not take my excuses. Upon opening the door to one, I had yet another supporter that did not allow me to slack off or feel sorry for myself. When I was caring for everyone else, Mr. Blanks was the other person pushing me to make myself a priority.

After a couple of years of training with him, I became confident in my physical needs and did not hesitate to try out different fitness classes. The experience of being a Drenched family member helped me in more ways than one. First, it helped me immensely with socialization. All of the people who attended the gym from all walks of life supported me. We were supportive of each other. Some of them even became great acquaintances that I continue to keep in contact with.

Being a gym member, I became a social butterfly, something I had not done since high school. This experience allowed me to care even better for myself and add more self-care things to my "to-do" list. Before you know it, I had my self-care routine, which included fitness, manicures and pedicures, facials, massages, acupuncture, and much more! The best part about it was that I did not feel guilty about treating myself well.

Now I have a question for you. As you read my real-life example of navigating self-care, did that sound like your story? Does the thought of sharing your story and being vulnerable frighten you to the point where you stare off somewhere and shut down? Does being able not to feel guilty about treating yourself seem too much like a fantasy to you because you're hard-wired in your ways or so used to how things usually are or how they've always been? This transformation from emotional turmoil to transforming into a person who socializes, doesn't have anxiety around others, and cannot only know what to do in their downtime but has a list of things to choose from is also available to you. This is not a unicorn story; it's your story, too; you just have to be willing and open to the possibility that this can be your story. That is what this book is all about, and together we will get you there.

SELF-CARE CHRONICLES

2020 was rough for us, and I was not an exception. I worked as an Emergency Room R.N.; my husband, a business owner, traveled extensively for work that we could not afford to turn down. I was incredibly stressed as we have two children, one of whom had trouble adjusting to the new normal. To make things worse, my manager was completely unsupportive. She would regularly deny me shift change requests needed to care for my children or respond to them when it was too late to make the change. I would have to leave them on their own for 14-hour stretches at a time. They would wake up after I left, and when I got home, it would be time for them to sleep. The public was scared and ungrateful, mad about exceedingly long waits. Our ER was overrun with patients who were sicker than they had ever been, and there were so many of them that we had patients in the hallway. Staff morale was down, and I was at a breaking point.

Syrenthia's Self-Care directives helped me put everything in perspective. She encouraged me to take time for myself and suggested I return to Zumba (online), as I love to dance. She insisted I carve out time to read as I am a voracious reader, and ultimately the I Care 4 Me First model had me set my boundaries at work. When management continued to fail to support me, I handed in my notice. Of course, after I gave my notice, they suddenly became super accommodating, but I had been practicing self-love, and I knew my value. I now work happily managing our business with hours that support my children's needs. I walked away from that madness and walked towards a better, realized life. Self-Care is not an option; it is a necessity like air and water and love. Let Syrenthia show you how to care for yourself first.

NIA TAYLOR-COLINO
BSN

CHAPTER 3

YOU NEED A SELF-CARE PLAN

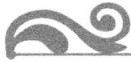

D o you know the feeling of a panic attack coming on? The feeling of being mentally or physically exhausted, overwhelmed, and stretched too thin. If you are looking for a reminder to take a break from working hard as a stay home parent or outside the home, this is it. Do not skip or neglect your basic needs. When you notice your sleep being affected, diet, lack of focus, feelings of low self-esteem, burnout, feeling unappreciated, and other negative ways, it is time to do something about it.

When you've been going nonstop and simply, need some alone time, staying in toxic friendships or relationships because you're scared of hurting someone else, and getting stuck in vicious cycles of going through the same motions daily, look into finding outlets. How often do you prioritize caring for yourself? Do you remember the last time you had some fun, relaxed, or just slowed things down? When was the last time you felt like yourself and worked on your dreams and passions? When you begin to notice that your priority list includes doing 80% for others and only 20% for you, you must gain compassion for yourself.

Self-care is a common topic lately, but it is often poorly explained. Perhaps you see it mentioned in self-help books or magazines and articles but do not clearly understand how you should add it to your life. As a result, it may appear wishy-washy or vague to you.

Alternatively, you may not be convinced that you simply should practice self-care regularly. You may think that your resources are better saved for working and taking care of others. So, let's discuss. What is self-care? And why is it vital?

WHAT IS SELF-CARE?

Self-care is a broad term that encompasses everything that we do. In a nutshell, it is about being as good to yourself as you would be to others. It is partly about knowing when your resources are running low and stepping back to replenish them instead of letting them all drain away. It also involves integrating self-compassion into your life in a way that helps to prevent the possibility of having burnout. It is important to remember that not everything that feels good is defined as self-care. We all can be tempted to utilize unhealthy coping mechanisms such as alcohol, drugs, over-eating, risk-taking, etc. These self-destructive activities assist us in managing challenging emotions, but the relief that we feel from these things is temporary. The distinction between unhealthy coping mechanisms and self-care activities is that the latter is an uncontroversial ideal for you. Self-care possesses long-term benefits for the mind and body when practiced correctly. Self-care is vital for our physical, emotional, and mental well-being. You should not neglect self-care, and here are some reasons why:

Know your worth: Self-care is necessary to maintain a healthy relationship with yourself as it creates positive feelings and boosts your confidence and self-esteem. Self-care is also vital to remind yourself and others that your needs are essential.

A healthy work-life balance: Contrary to popular belief, workaholism is not a virtue. Overwork, and the accompanying stress paired with exhaustion, can lead to lesser productivity and a disorganized and emotionally depleted you. It could also result in health problems, from anxiety and depression to insomnia and heart diseases. Professional self-care habits such as taking intermittent breaks (for lunch, calling your mom, or taking a stroll), avoiding overextending yourself, and setting professional boundaries allow you to stay sharp, motivated, and healthier.

Stress management: While a small dose of stress is a healthy way to give us the nudge that we require to meet the deadlines or finish overdue tasks, constant stress and anxiety can significantly affect your mental and physical health. Smart self-care habits such as eating healthy, connecting with a beloved, or practicing meditation reduce the toxic effects of stress by enhancing your mood, boosting your energy, and increasing your confidence levels.

Start living, stop existing: Life is a sweet gift. Why waste it when we possess the choice to live a more meaningful existence? Yes, you may have a lot of responsibilities, but it is vital to remember that taking care of yourself is also your responsibility. In fact, it is your main responsibility. Little things like sipping tea while watching the raindrops racing down the window pane, enjoying a hot bubble bath, or reading your favorite book are ideas that are necessary for your day to day happiness. Doing things like taking up a new hobby or learning a new language can make your life more purposeful by presenting you with new reasons to wake up in the mornings.

Better physical health: Self-care is not solely about your mental health. It is also about caring for your physical self by eating healthy, caring about your hygiene, receiving adequate sleep, and exercising regularly.

TYPES OF SELF-CARE

One of the main excuses people make for ignoring books about self-care is that they just do not have time. The great news is that there are many various self-care practices, and none of them are especially difficult or require too much planning. The trick is to seek out things you genuinely enjoy that fit with your life and values. Once you start adding emotional self-care to your life, you are likely to become fiercely protective of that time. You will also often wonder how you ever managed in the absence of it.

Here are the five primary categories of self-care:

Spiritual
Getting in touch with God, your inner being, true values, and what really matters to you.

Physical
Physical activity is important for your body and well-being and it is instrumental in assisting you in letting off steam.

Sensory

When you are able to tune into the details of the sensations around you by using your five senses, it becomes easier to live in the present moment. When you are in the present, you can more effectively let go of resentments related to the past or anxieties about the future.

Emotional

Ensure you are fully engaged with your emotions. When you face them head-on, it helps with stress. You may feel tempted to push down feelings like sadness or anger, but it is healthy to feel them, accept them, and move on. You are not blameworthy for your emotions, only how you respond to them. Remember that emotions are not "good" or "bad" in themselves.

Social

Social self-care might look different depending on whether you are introverted or extroverted. However, connecting with other people is essential for happiness. It helps you to understand that you are not alone. It can also give us a sense of being fully "seen" by others. This can help us fight loneliness and isolation. Social self-care is not about just doing *things* with others but choosing to do something meaningful with people you care about and make you feel good.

WHY DO WE NEED A SELF-CARE PLAN?

The right self-care plan can help improve your well-being, assist with stress management, and help maintain your health. It is easy to let taking care of yourself fall to the bottom of your list when life gets crazy. It is always the first thing we sacrifice because it does not seem as important as the other things we deal with daily in the midst of chaos. We end up substituting our important self-care things for the urgent things way more than we should. After a while, it starts to require a lot out of our lives through exhaustion, burnout, decreased focus, lack of motivation, and more. Whatever the case may be, it is necessary to spend a little time getting to know yourself and what your mind, body, and soul need to function at your highest level. By learning to spot activities and things that support your well-being, you will be ready to create a customized self-care plan that works specifically for you.

How to Create a Self-Care Plan

The first step in making your self-care plan is to create a list of the things you value and need every day, like reading with a cup of coffee in the morning, walking with your dog, or taking an evening yoga class. To layer on to that, consider the items you do not necessarily want to experience daily. Try to focus on the things that cause you to be happy and spiritually fulfilled. Of course, things like getting a manicure and pedicure are often on your self-care plan, but attempt to think more outside the box. Try learning a different hobby, checking your closet to discard belongings you do not need, or finally making that dreaded commitment to wash out your pantry. One of my favorite daily checklist items is to select one thing that has been on my mental "to-do" list and get it taken care of. This one is surprisingly very satisfying.

Consider your self-care plan on a daily and weekly basis. Make time at least three days per week to do it for yourself. It helps you to brainstorm about practices or activities within the following seven different categories or "domains" of life:

Financial: make a budget for the present and future income that you plan to receive; handle taxes and other financial responsibilities; gain an overall understanding of how finances will affect current (and future) decisions

Social: invest in healthy relationships; schedule time to spend time with people who interest you; be intentional about making phone calls to those you care for; remain conscious of people's birthdays; prioritize important events

Professional: chase work-life balance; invest in new skills; set boundaries; network; work on time management skills; plan for the future

Emotional: seek feedback from others; reason with and express yourself; journal about your feelings; express thoughts and emotions with others; invest time in positive activities; monitor self-talk; take advantage of great thoughts; celebrate achievements

Physical: take care of your physical body; eat well; exercise; get adequate rest; attend doctor's appointments; moisturize; get proper nutrients.

Psychological: journal; set personal goals; learn new skills; spend time alone; self-reflect; brain dump when experiencing mental and emotional overloads

Spiritual: attend church and small groups; invest in the community and get involved; spend time reading devotionals and scriptures; turn off the radio in the car to spend time praying; start each day with prayer; meditate on scripture

Consider how you are currently taking care of yourself in these areas, then think about ways you could improve and add things you would wish to try. Of course, some areas will prove to be more critical than others, but you want to consider how you are addressing each category. On a daily basis, you want to prioritize your physical needs just as much as you are taking care of your professional and psychological needs. Adding more balance into our day-to-day routine will assist your productivity and total well-being. It will also enable you to be more resilient when life gets stressful. Once you have an inventory of things that contribute positively to your physical, spiritual, and emotional needs, it is time to place your plan into action.

The key is to yield a conscious effort and investment in yourself. By putting things that contribute to your self-care into writing, you commit to putting your happiness and well-being first. And that is something we all need to do a little more of.

What does your self-care plan look like? Take a moment with a piece of paper and a pen or a pencil and commit that to writing right now. There is no time like the present to make this decision and commitment to care for yourself then right now.

SELF-CARE CHRONICLES

When Syrenthia asked me to write a testimonial for her new book, I was highly honored as I hold her in the highest regard. Here's my story. I own my own Bookkeeping business and have been her bookkeeper for a few years now. I have never met anyone like Syrenthia before – and I've worked with quite a few people from all walks of life. From the first introductory call, I knew she was someone special. Her positive energy and almost Zen-like calm leaps out of her, and you can't help but be affected by her energy. I personally have a lot going on. You could say I'm a bit "gimpy" and have a laundry list of ailments and surgeries. I try not to go into too much detail where my clients are concerned, but I told her my whole medical history on the first phone call – before she even hired me. I felt so relaxed talking to her, and we hit it off right away. She shared with me her history, and I just couldn't believe how upbeat she was for all that she has going on. I was diagnosed with Multiple Sclerosis 7 years ago and then had a cancer diagnosis six years ago. I've tried to change my mindset and values each day. I have pain daily but have been learning to take it one day at a time and find the positive in each day, and Syrenthia has strengthened this practice for me.

I had never heard the term "self-care" before. I always just called it a "me" day. When I heard her use this term, I adopted it right away, and I seem to use it all the time with my friends and family. The term self-care has so much power behind it. I tend to take on too many hats for my family, friends, and clients. I'm a people pleaser, and I realized that I was not taking care of myself in the same manner, and that was an eye-opening experience for me. She enforced the idea that you are no good to anyone else if you are not centered and calm.

Syrenthia has such an amazing attitude even when the world tries to push her down. She gets right on up and manages each day with grace and gratitude. On a particularly horrible, pain-riddle day, she happened to call and asked how I was doing. Well, let me tell you, the flood gates opened, and I went on an angry tirade about all my pain and how everything basically "sucked." I cannot believe I did that with a client, but I also consider her my friend. She "talked me off the ledge," so to speak, and reminded me to breathe and be grateful for what I have and that tomorrow is another day. She asked me if I had been practicing "self-care" lately, and I had not. I made a point to stop what I was working on and get some distance and just "be." I was not centered at all, and her pointing that out did wonders for me.

As a Bookkeeper and Business Owner, I tend to have crazy deadlines but have made a point to take time out for myself – no matter how busy I am – and do you know what? It has helped me more than I can say. I wake up every day, even the days when my whole body hurts, and I am just grateful to be alive. I believe that people enter our lives for a reason, and boy did she come at the perfect time in my life. I have been much more centered and calmer since meeting her. My goal is to have the same amount of inner peace that my friend Syrenthia has. I am lucky to have met her. I cannot wait for you all to read her book and work towards self-care and inner peace.

DENEEN MICHLAP
Owner/Bookkeeper
On The Dot Bookkeeping, Inc

CHAPTER 4

EMOTIONAL SELF-CARE

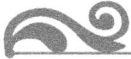

Unhealed emotional wounds create unhealthy strongholds in the mind.

You've arrived at the book chapter that was the most challenging to write. It's the longest chapter of the book, and not only was it a tricky topic for me to discuss but also one that is often harder to understand than anything else in this book. When discussing the many themes in this chapter, I thought about how deeply imprinted my view of the world was and people's overall perspective when talking about emotions. We all know that some emotions are "good" and others are "bad," but how does that contribute to how we see the world, how we see ourselves within the world?

How does it manifest itself in other aspects of our care? For example, how does it shape our mental self-care, physical self-care, and the different categories that we talked about in the previous chapter? Also, what work needs to be done to overcome those challenges that emotions can present?

That is what we are going to be tackling in this specific chapter. I ask that you do not gloss over this chapter with the eagerness to get to the end of this book. This chapter is in the middle of the book because that is where we often get lost, or that is where we get stuck with no hope of getting out—the middle. We will go deep in this chapter, but the reward will pay off for years and years to come, so let us jump two feet in.

When we talk about emotional self-care, it's important to realize there are many facets to it. It is chewy, like eating warm chocolate chip cookies without any milk to wash them down. The trials of life will have you down and leave you with no type of outlet to heal or escape. This leads to the temptation of abandoning our emotions altogether, which leaves us open to 3 areas that I struggled with:

1. Codependency
2. Self-Forgiveness
3. Emotional Trauma

I'll start with codependency. Researcher Darlene Lancer characterizes a codependent person as a person who belongs to a one-sided relationship where one person relies on the other to meet nearly all of their emotional and self-esteem needs. Another way you can look at codependency is a relationship that allows another person to maintain their irresponsible, addictive, or underachieving behavior. When you're in one of these relationships, you can find yourself pleasing people, having poor boundaries (more in chapter 5 about this), having low self-esteem, and lack of self-control.

Barbara De Angelis had this to say about codependency, "In all codependent relationships, the rescuer needs the victim as much as the rescuer." Can you feel the weight of that quote and the bondage that it can bring to your life? There is an attachment that comes with codependency that will bind you. This is how you can lose your identity. You fall into its web and then don't know how to get out.

Brokenness and emotional wounds then follow by putting limitations on your value and bringing emotional trauma into your life. My emotional trauma and neglect from early childhood were the root cause of why I looked for co-dependent love in people and things. It served as a distraction from my unhealed pain. When your identity is wrapped up in feeling needed by helping, rescuing, or enabling another person's addiction, which could be caused by, poor emotional health, immaturity, irresponsibility, or underachievement, then you are essentially under arrest by the spirit of codependency. I got to the point where I was no longer a fixer of other people's emotional darkness while looking over myself. Emotional trauma is an experience that I need to learn to go through and forgive.

Have you ever felt like forgiving someone felt like a piece of cake while forgiving yourself, on the other hand, felt wrong and unfair? Research has shown that individuals who practice the art of **self-forgiveness** have been said to have better lives, mental states, and emotional well-being. When you seek to forgive yourself, you approach yourself with kindness and mercy just as you would do another human being. To work on actively forgiving yourself at all times, you must remain mindful. By being mindful, you become aware. By becoming aware, you actively analyze your actions to ensure that you act rationally. It is also important to practice compassion. Everyone we meet is fighting a silent battle that we are unaware of. By practicing compassion with others, you will begin to show yourself the same kindness. Give yourself time, take care of yourself, and tend to your needs. Ensure that you are putting yourself first to not live in a sorry state. Dr. Carole Pertofsky stated, "Learning to be self-forgiving is a skill that requires practice. Over time, you will notice that you are more relaxed, open, and happy. You will be able to notice and appreciate how much pleasure can be found in a simple moment, how much there is to be grateful for in everyday life, and how much the world needs you and your special gifts and talents."

Emotional trauma occurs when extraordinary stressful events come into our lives to shake up our current sense of self. Emotional trauma can cause you to feel like you are on edge all of the time, angry, disconnected, numb, and often unable to trust anyone. Emotional trauma can be caused by ongoing stress, overlooked issues growing into more significant problems, or one-time events. A few more symptoms of emotional trauma include insomnia, fatigue, muscle tension, anxiety, edginess, and agitation. Regardless of what has happened in your life, it is important to know that things will get better. You will heal and move forward. Try going outside and exercising to get yourself out of your emotional funk. Also, consider joining small groups or social clubs in your community. Furthermore, take care of your health and get plenty of rest. Finally, find someone you can confide in when you feel like emotional trauma is taking over your life.

I had to learn to work through codependency, emotional trauma, and the struggle with forgiving myself to finally move forward into the future that my Higher Power had for me. Because I am harder on myself than I am on anyone else, I had to put in extra work to forgive myself so that I could heal emotionally.

Prayer for Emotional Healing:
Heavenly Father, forgive me for using distractions as a form of healing. I am in agreement with you to continue working on my emotional healing day in and day out.

How often do you hear people say they don't know where to start when it comes to healing? I can speak from personal experience that it is expected when you are carrying around years of trauma and pain from your past that has not been dealt with. Not setting healthy boundaries was a struggle in my personal life, which caused me to carry around other people's baggage. To heal, I was willing to set firm boundaries to make some significant changes. Having a great mentor, a great vessel from my higher power, GOD, helps me restore my faith.

My emotional healing began with a deep cleansing of the spirits I battled with for many years; codependency and victimization. Both come from my family system and emotionally controlled others. The two had me searching for what I was missing from my parents, who played a role in releasing my emotional trauma. These spirits controlled me in ways that were not healthy for me. I attracted people with my parent's mannerisms in all my relationships, whether family, friendships, or business. All relationships mirror their emotional trauma. As I share my healing, I am filled with gratitude, knowing that my parents, who did not play a mental or emotional role in my life growing up, have played a massive role in my healing.

Fifteen years ago, I met my mentor at a family friend's house. Little did I know, my Heavenly Father had introduced me to the vessel, my sister in Christ, who would assist me on my emotional healing journey.

My healing started with writing down all the things I needed to work on for myself. The top of my list included the codependency and victimization spirits. As I began to work on my list, I realized how I shifted from being codependent and a victim. By being 50/50 of both, I was emotionally controlled by both my parents and the individual I attracted that had the exact characteristics of my parents. I was blind to see how they would spend the time, effort, and money, giving and taking from the other.

Establishing boundaries within relationships was a challenge. With my family, I felt that I was obligated to support them financially. Friends that were considered family members also drained me mentally and emotionally. In business relationships, I made all of the deposits and rarely saw any returns from them. There were no boundaries when it came to my relationships. I allowed all 3 of my relationships to deplete my emotional gas tank. I was giving to the takers and receiving nothing in return but anger within myself for not setting any type of boundaries.

As I worked on myself and my healing, I became honest with myself and others. Setting boundaries and caring for my inner being became my top priority. I would never change the nice person I am, but surely I do not want to be distracted by people who are not at peace. Peace is such a wonderful feeling, and without it, you open the doors to distractions and disturbance. When I sense a distraction coming along, I instantly set the tone for our relationship, not the relationship setting the tone for me. I am mindful of the words I speak and the energy I receive. I am always in a positive mood from when I wake up to going to bed at night. I don't take things personally because life is what you make it to be. I refuse to let anyone squeeze me into their mold. Setting boundaries played a massive part in healing me. I did the work I needed to do to forgive myself and rid myself of toxic relationships, whether family, friends, or business.

THE RESULTS FROM THE WORK

Once I became a mother, I made a point to be present physically, mentally, and emotionally, not just financially, for my kids. My greatest accomplishment in this lifetime is succeeding in the wonderful job of raising my loving son on the autism spectrum and an amazing daughter with a pure heart. I can't forget my bonus children: my youngest daughter, who became mine at 14 years old, and another son at 23 years old. It is a beautiful site to see them as the loving, caring, and emotionally fulfilled young adults they are today.

I believe everyone on the journey towards self-care ultimately desires those they care for and love to be well while not at the expense of their well-being. That is what happened to me and why I'm confident you, too, can experience this for yourself. Now I know that it is easier said than done. It's said that only in the dictionary does the word "success" come before "work," which is the truth with your self-care journey. However, some work will need to be done, and I'm about to share with you the tools that it takes to get there with my 4 "PPPT" tools.

These tools are a part of my daily self-care routine, which consists of my morning spiritual meditation, fitness, and self-affirmations. Each day I have is one I do not take for granted, so I approach it as the blessing it is and operate from my purpose and intention.

THE 4 PPPT TOOLS

Peace: How do you maintain your peace in your day? Starting the day with prayers, devotionals, and conversations with My GOD.

Patience: What or who tests your patience? If you run into a situation where someone or something is testing your patience, you have to check in with your higher self quickly. How would you handle it? Take a step back, and don't be quick to make poor judgments. Go straight into a conversation with words of wisdom.

Protection: How do you protect yourself throughout the day? Before my day gets started, I have meditated with prayers and scriptures. Further, I silently sit with my eyes closed and listen to the universe.

Trust: What or how do you work on your trust for the day? Practicing your faith in God each day allows God's powerful words to fill you with trust and understanding.

It is by practicing with these four tools that I can care for my nine spirits, what is also referred to as the fruits of the spirits:

CARING FOR MY 9 SPIRITS

1. Self-control
2. Gentleness
3. Faithfulness
4. Goodness
5. Kindness
6. Patience
7. Peace
8. Joy
9. Love

You can expect to see yourself growing in these nine specific areas when doing the work.

Before we conclude this chapter on emotional self-care, there are a few more things. One is the two primary ways I've observed myself and other people handle their feelings regarding emotional self-care. What lies at the core of both of them is recognizing the validity of your emotional state. You undeniably benefit from accepting how you are feeling right now, and this is something that is already happening anyway. Any plan to hide what you are feeling from yourself can only bring additional tension. It is, of course, easier to accept some feelings over others. We usually do not have a drag embracing the resonance of peace, excitement, happiness, love, or gratitude. But, we would like to make a conscious effort to welcome sadness, anger, anxiety, impatience, or regret. In my opinion, making this effort is the foundation of emotional self-care. Once you have recognized and (hopefully) accepted how you are emotional, there are two ways to go about it: you either attempt to alter your spirit (emotional state) or choose not to. You decide to change your circumstances to impact the way you feel.

MENTAL SELF-CARE

Thoughts in our heads can cause a mess, especially if we do not notice them. Sometimes we drift away in our thoughts, usually the most anxiety-ridden ones, and after half an hour, we cannot even tell what we have been brooding over. All we know is that we are left with feelings of discomfort. Why is this the case?

Mental self-care is a two-fold process for me:

The first step is to consistently analyze my thoughts and why I am even thinking certain things. As soon as I manage to take stock of my thoughts, they cannot direct my life. The second step is acquiring those mental habits and beliefs that serve me in the highest forms. This can be done after observing my thought content for a short duration. By doing so, I can tell which mental habits nurture my well-being and which do not.

It is worth noting that some mental habits are way more beneficial for you than others. Therefore, cultivating healthy habits is the second step in developing great mental self-care. I believe that this is what some Buddhist traditions refer to when they speak about creating more positive impressions in our minds. According to my personal experiences, these "positive impressions" include:

- Practicing gratitude throughout each day

- Exercising patience over being in a hurry to get things done
- Focusing your attention on the present moment
- Practicing acceptance of what is already happening

PHYSICAL SELF-CARE

This aspect of self-care is the most candid, and it comes down to making sure that your body is well-nourished and happy. Three essential elements of physical self-care include good nutrition, a sufficient amount of recovery time (rest and sleep), and necessary exercise. After you begin to take care of your physical self, you might have other ways to care for your body depending on your preferences and state of health. For example, your actions could lead to long baths, massages, physiotherapy, breathing exercises, etc. I cherish the metaphor that refers to the body as your "real home," "temple," or "vehicle." Your body is the only constant that you have throughout your entire life.

Given that you only have one body, you want to ensure it functions as well as possible so that you can enjoy every experience. You should also approach caring for your physical body holistically. Your body is a system that functions as one. You cannot just take care of your arms and skip the legs. You cannot say that your back pain is a problem separated from everything else but claim that your smoking habit does not have anything to do with that. But, of course, it does. Everything in your body is connected. Moreover, it is also connected to the things happening inside your head.

When it involves physical self-care, ask yourself these subsequent questions to assess whether there could be some areas that you would like to improve:

Is your current diet fueling your body well?
Are you taking charge of your health?
Are you getting adequate sleep at night?
Are you getting enough exercise during the week?
Why is emotional self-care so important?

Now that we know about our emotional self-care, it is time that we dive into the thing that will put us at the most significant risk of all, our relationship with boundaries.

SELF-CARE CHRONICLES

I'm grateful to have a friend like Syrenthia. I looked up to her as a role model for balancing work life and family and being a caregiver by always advocating Self-care since the first day I met her 13 years ago. I've been an active Realtor for 17 years which can be very stressful, and I take care of my one and only sibling, my brother, who, after my mom passed away nine years ago was left to my care.

One of the joys of being a Realtor is meeting new people that I get to help with their goals, and Syrenthia was one of them. Not only did I work with her, we have become friends and her family has become family and she has always been a great example of someone who practices what she preaches... so when I would get her advice and receive her reminders on how to take care of yourself first....I trusted her. She would invite me to get facials, salt baths, massages, which I would do occasionally, but after seeing her continue doing these things since I've met her, I knew that I might need to follow her example. I started to get regular facials because of her and regularly get massages. She made sure we knew she prioritized taking time to take care of herself first, knowing she took that time but still could work hard, care for her friends and a big family, and be a caregiver for her son....it was apparent she was doing something right. Things like that were something I would only do occasionally, and prioritizing my clients and business was on top of my list. And not until I realized that when I slacked on practicing self-care routines, especially during the beginning of the pandemic, where, for example, I paused going to the gym, ate a lot of comfort food, and in turn, gained a lot of unwanted weight....I realized my inner peace was deteriorating and would take my stress out on my loved ones. And after learning the hard way, I realized what Syrenthia has been preaching to us....should be a way of life and incorporated into our daily practice. And now that I had a minor setback or "learned the hard way" after a breakup, I realized the importance of self-care and taking the time to be alone...and that it is a "practice." And thankfully, I have friends like Syrenthia, who constantly reminds us to be kind to ourselves, take care of ourselves first, and remove the harmful or toxic things from our lives so we can be happier, which makes other people around us more comfortable. With a career like mine, and having to care for my brother....I make sure to prioritize things like meditating, allowing myself to feel and journal, exercise, and keep my mind, body and soul as best as I can with what I can control. I'm grateful for having Syrenthia to turn to for positive advice and receiving her daily suggestions for self care... because I know she lives it...and it shows.

JENNIFER CAYENTO SALLAVE,
Realtor

SETTING HEALTHY BOUNDARIES

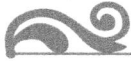

D o you know what serves as life's mirror more than anything else? Relationships! When you look in a mirror, you look to see what you look like, which is what relationships do. Relationships help you discover who you are. But like a real-life mirror, it does not stop there. You are able to see things that need to be addressed and relationships do that too. Relationships also teach us a thing or two. They show us the people we are attracted to and also the people we need to stay away from too. That is where boundaries come into play.

Before we dive into healthy boundaries allow me to define what they are. The author of the best-selling book, "Boundaries", Henry Cloud says this about boundaries, "Boundaries define us. They define what is me and what is not me. A boundary shows me where I end and where someone else begins." Boundaries are crucial when we talk about healthy relationships, and no not just with others, with ourselves too.

I learned to set boundaries with family members, friends, and in my personal and business relationships. A relationship is just that; a relationship where the most common rules are communication, consideration, compassion, love and most of all boundaries. When you don't set those boundaries, you will find yourself stressed out and taking things out on yourself because you didn't set the right tone with boundaries initially.

Boundaries are not optional. They are necessary if you want to focus, achieve your own goals, and reach your standard of success. Personal boundaries are the bounds that you decide to work for you. They are standards that you can set on how people can treat you, how they will behave around you, and what they will expect from you. They are drawn from the framework of your core beliefs, perspective, experiences, opinions, and values.

If you do not set healthy boundaries, you are likely to be at the mercy of others. It also means that you will take away time and energy for yourself to do what others want you to do. Eventually, this will cause frustration and depression because you may start to feel disappointed and lost. Boundaries serve many functions. They help to guard us, clarify our responsibilities, preserve our physical and emotional energies, and help us to spot our limits according to our beliefs and values.

Signs that you lack boundaries?

Two words: guilt and anxiety.

Have you ever felt responsible if others were not happy? If someone is having a bad day, you wonder or feel it had something to do with you or something you did or did not do. Many individuals with boundary issues feel guilty for the smallest of things. It can be as simple as taking the last piece of cake or asking someone to give you a little space on a bench so that you too can sit. While these may look super small, do you notice anything about it? Who is the person that always ends up with the shortest end of the stick, or even worse, who is the person often left out? The person who feels guilty for speaking up and saying what they want and need.

If speaking up for yourself causes you anxiety or you've found yourself on the side of saying yes all of the time, it is a sign that you may be lacking boundaries. The fear of disappointing someone because you made a decision that was best for you should not contribute to the stress we feel daily. What is the cost of letting this guilt, fear, and anxiety make the decisions for us? We then are left wondering who we are. Are the decisions you make you or the people you are so fearful of.

Here is something to think about... always doing what others want puts you in a position where you are left to cram time into your life. Remember those days of cramming for a test? Typically something gets forgotten when you do so, and in this case, for us caregivers, those others rely upon the most, what gets forgotten is us. As a result, we are left with the exhaustion of putting everyone else's fires at the expense of our fire.

If you are looking for an energy boost, the answer may not be a 5-hour energy drink; the answer might just be you setting boundaries. I've found that setting boundaries energize me. The same can happen with you when you put the fear, guilt, and anxiety to the side and intentionally put things in place to protect and care for you.

Here are a few other mile makers that can help you identify if your boundaries could use a little adjusting:

- You find decision-making a real challenge.
- Your radar is off when it comes to sharing.
- You are constantly the victim of situations.

As I shared earlier, victimization can show up a lot on your self-care journey. Unfortunately, many who fall into victimization will often not even realize it is happening. That is the scariest part of it all and is why an entire chapter is being dedicated to this. An entire book could be written on this alone. One has been written and is a New York Times bestseller. It's worth reading as you further your personal development in this specific area of self-care.

IDENTIFYING YOUR LIMITS

The first step in setting boundaries is getting clear about your bounds—emotional, mental, physical, and spiritual. You do this by paying attention to yourself, noticing what you can tolerate and accept, and what makes you feel uncomfortable and stressed.

These feelings will assist you in clarifying your limits.

PAY ATTENTION TO YOUR FEELINGS

There are three essential feelings that are usually red flags or cues that you need to either set boundaries in a particular situation or that you are not maintaining your boundaries:

1. **Discomfort**

2. **Resentment**
3. **Guilt**

You can visualize these feelings as cues to yourself that a boundary issue may be present. If a specific situation, person, or area of your life leads you to feel uncomfortable, resentful, or guilty, and it has happened many times, this is often a crucial cue. For instance, resentment usually develops from feelings of being taken advantage of or not being appreciated. In addition, it is often a sign that you simply are extending yourself beyond your limits because you are feeling guilty and want to be considered an honest parent, spouse, sibling, child, friend, or employee. Another common contributor is someone attempting to impose their expectations, beliefs, or values on you.

Boundaries are designed to guard you and your overall well-being. It is often helpful to consider these feelings on a continuum to determine whether a boundary may have to be set. When a situation occurs, ask yourself, "How uncomfortable, resentful, or guilty am I feeling?" Your answer should be rated on a scale of 1-10 (10 being the highest). If your level of discomfort happens to be at a 3, consider this within the lower zone and having a light effect on your emotions. Ratings of 4 to 6 are within the medium zone, indicating a more significant impact on you. Scores between 7 and 10 are considered the high zone, and a boundary should be set immediately.

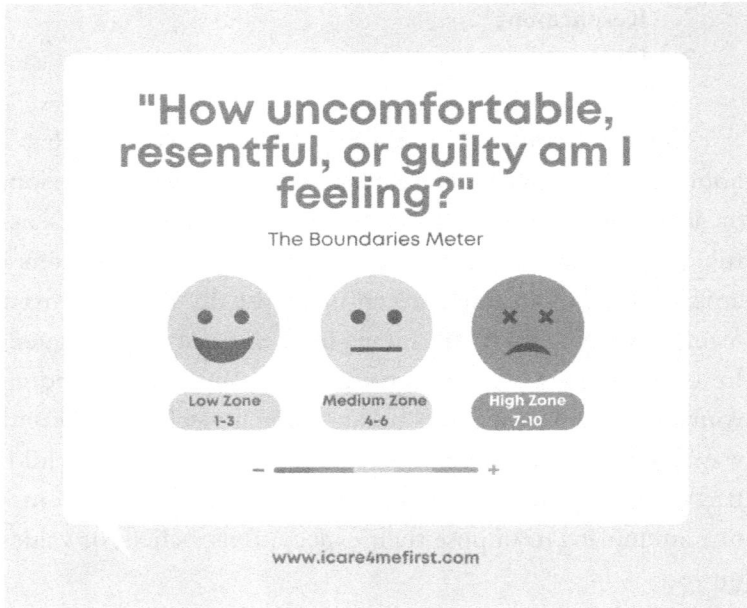

"How uncomfortable, resentful, or guilty am I feeling?"

The Boundaries Meter

Low Zone 1-3 · Medium Zone 4-6 · High Zone 7-10

www.icare4mefirst.com

GIVE YOURSELF PERMISSION TO SET BOUNDARIES

The biggest obstacles often experienced at some point when setting boundaries are the feelings of fear, guilt, and self-doubt. Never feel bad about how people will respond (e.g., angry, hurt) if you set and enforce your boundaries. Do not feel guilty about speaking up about your feelings or saying no to a loved one. Often, people feel like they ought to be ready to deal with a situation and say yes based on what an honest sibling, friend, or spouse would do. Don't worry. You may question whether you have the proper boundaries set at first. When these doubts occur, reaffirm that you have the right to set boundaries, permit yourself, and work to keep them.

CONSIDER YOUR ENVIRONMENT

The environment you are in serves as your context and can strongly influence your behaviors, attitudes, and perceptions. Family and work environments are two examples of powerful contexts and social circles. You may be wondering, why is it important to think about your environment when it involves setting boundaries? Your environment can either support the boundaries, making it less challenging for you, or present obstacles to boundary setting, making things more difficult. For example, consider your social circle of close friends. Are these relationships generally reciprocal, with a natural give and take? Or, do they feel unbalanced with you more often giving than you receive? Always be mindful of who you share your energy. If the relationships are unstable, you will feel more uncomfortable, making things more challenging for you to set and maintain boundaries.

ALWAYS STAND BY YOUR WORDS

The most significant part of having boundaries is how you communicate them. You can possess the most healthy set of boundaries, but if they are not displayed clearly, you will build some confusing relationships for yourself and everyone else. One way to quickly get someone to question your character or authenticity is by saying one thing and doing another. Sometimes we are scared to confront others with the truth in love and other relationships. We hide our true feelings in exchange for being concerned about other people's feelings and reactions. I've learned that the more you ground yourself with your boundaries and values, the more you will be ready to be firm in your communication.

What boundaries will you begin to put in place to better care for yourself? Make a list of the people, the environments, and commitments that you are not willing to budge on. Your boundaries will either set you free, or the lack will imprison you. The choice is yours.

SELF-CARE CHRONICLES

Self-care is hard for me. I admit it. I can barely get to my doctor appointments between school pickup, deadlines at work, and all the sports practices and games on our family's schedule. So you probably won't find me at the spa on Tuesday afternoon. However, I have learned so much from Syrenthia, and I have her to thank for even the small moments I take for myself.

I wondered how she did it, how she took on so many responsibilities with such grace and dedication, and how she remained calm in circumstances that would drive others mad. Then, through her work with POCWASN and iCare4Me-First, she revealed her superpower. Self-care. She truly supports and nurtures herself in the same way she cares for those closest to her.

At first, I thought that may sound selfish. However, I've witnessed how that principal has had the opposite effect on Syrenthia's life and the lives of those around her. When she feels whole and fulfilled, she can show up as the best mother, wife, sister, daughter, and friend that she can be. You can feel the calm in her home as soon as you walk in, and I truly believe it begins with her inner peace.

CiCi has gently reminded me, on many occasions, that it's not really a superpower. It is an attainable goal that we can all work towards on a small or large scale. Her work in the community and commitment to sharing the gift she has discovered, is such a testament to it working.

As a young mother, I struggled to find myself after having my boys. I felt like I needed to give everything I had to my family. I made changes in my career, hobbies, and relationships to be more available as "mom." But over time, my selflessness began breeding resentment and I knew I had to make a change. I have not mastered the art as well as Mrs. Colino, but I started small and felt a shift almost immediately.

I now try to get better sleep to rest and recover my body. I speak kindly to and about myself. I read more and enjoy the quiet times, to expand my knowledge and challenge my beliefs. I try to move daily with a workout or a walk outside to remind myself I am powerful. And just by setting realistic expectations in the workplace and home, I have felt an improvement in my overall happiness. I recognize we are all in different seasons of our lives, and self-care looks different because of that; but Syrenthia has shown me through her actions alone, that self-care works and it is important for all of us. I will continue to work on myself and encourage other mothers and caretakers to do the same. I am forever grateful to CiCi for showing me the value in myself, and letting me accept it in my own time.

MEGAN BULOW
Accountant

CHAPTER 6

SELF-CARE MINDSET

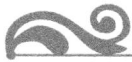

S elf-care involves planning for and truly taking the time to tend to your basic physical, mental, and emotional needs. It is the conscious rest which assists you and recharges your batteries. It is the time when you are the most present through life's simple pleasures. It is your ability to stop, smile inwardly, and ask yourself: "How are you doing today? What do you need?" Then, it is attending to those needs with an enormous dose of kindness, compassion, patience, and love.

Self-care is not just one specific activity.

Self-care is a mindset; a dedication to addressing and prioritizing personal wants and needs. Self-care can be as simple as remembering to take care of yourself with the same level of importance you would place on those you care for like a spouse, partner, kids, or a friend. We are all unique individuals. The things we desire regarding self-care differ among us and self-care routines can change throughout an individual's life.

Self-care includes taking intentional time daily to tend to your needs (not your chores); exercise, have fun, spend time with others, or spend time with yourself. While this may seem out of reach for some, setting aside a small amount of time a few days a week is a great beginning. Make a simple list of things you can do to assist in shaping your mind for self-care and watch how it grows.

To assist you in coming together with your own plan of self-care I'd like to share with you some tips that can help you in developing your self-care mindset. Some of these tips specifically share what deviates one from implementing their own self-care plan and others will specifically give you practical things you can do right now to start slowly and surely building your self-care castle brick by brick.

Tips for Developing Your Self-Care Mindset

1. Stop comparing yourself to others

One of the nicest gifts you can give to yourself is making the decision to stop comparing yourself to others. When you are constantly comparing yourself to other people and feeling like you do not stack up, you are discounting your own uniqueness and taking away any chance of being happy with who you are. Developing your self-care mindset entails learning how to be proud of who you are no matter how you see people, or how people see you. This is especially true if you are comparing yourself to the people you see on social media. All you are seeing is a snapshot of one moment in time. Remember that you only see what people want you to see. You do not see all the hard work and struggle behind the scenes of the lives of others.

2. Include a morning workout in your self-care plan

One of the first things to fall by the wayside when you are not taking care of yourself is your fitness routine. It is so easy to say "I do not have time for the gym" or "I will stop on the way home." Changing your self-care mindset to include time for exercise is important for your physical, mental, and emotional well-being. It is the most unique gift you can give yourself, not only because it will improve your physical health, but you will also find yourself feeling better and more accomplished after you are done too.

I personally recommend working out first thing in the mornings. This has helped me in so many ways. If you exercise in the mornings, you are sure to get it done and the post-exercise endorphins will give you a lift throughout the rest of the day. Even if you cannot get to the gym in the mornings, try to carve out some time for a walk or jog around the neighborhood. It is usually the quietest time of the day and you can even combine walking and meditation as a way to get both self-care suggestions into your routine.

3. Learn to say no

One of the most enormous changes you will need to make when developing a self-care mindset is learning to say no to others. Saying no is among the most important aspects of self-care. When you say no, you learn to honor yourself by showing respect for your time. If you cannot do a project or a favor, say no. Do not add stress to your life just to be accommodating to someone else. Accommodate you first. Learning to say no can be empowering. People will learn how to respect your boundaries and your time. Moreover, it allows you to have additional time to focus on your self-care.

4. Take time to meditate and reflect.

A few minutes of meditation or quiet reflection a day can be soothing to the soul. As little as five minutes of quiet time upon rising in the morning can help remind you that your self-care is vital. The best part about meditation is that the longer you do it, the better it gets. Start with five minutes each day and work your way up to twenty. Adding meditation to your self-care practice helps you to relieve stress and leaves you feeling way better afterward.

5. Try something out of your comfort zone.

This does not have to be skydiving or bungee jumping (however that would be pretty cool, too), but maybe make a new friend or introduce yourself to a new group within your community. Look for things that you can do where you do not know anyone to have room to meet new people or do a Facebook live to connect with all those hundreds of friends you have! Every time we challenge our comfort zone, it grows, and soon those things that used to scare us become part of our daily lives.

6. Un-plug.

If you can (and there are some legit reasons why some people cannot), turn off your cell phone or put it on the "DO NOT DISTURB" mode at night. Try to keep your phone cut off overnight if you can. Being constantly reachable can affect your mental state. Not to mention, the distraction of constant notifications can easily cause you to experience burnout. Remember, you do not have to be everything to everyone at all times. Take some time for yourself.

These are just some of the tips that I've seen work for me and the many people I've had conversations with through my time as a caregiver, running my organizations geared towards caring for yourself. There are many more that you can read about in the resources section of this book which will link you to more tips that you can use. This journey is a life-long one. Thus no one book could include all the tips. However, add to the fact that self-care is different for each individual. You will realize that being present and conscious, as we talked about in the opening paragraph of this chapter, is one of the best ways to develop a strategy and game plan that works specifically for you and one that you will maintain, scale, and grow as you grow into the best version of you.

To help jumpstart you, here are a few questions that I want you to ponder.

How can you function from a healthy self-care mindset? This question helps us to think not about our trauma or past but more about the possibilities of our future. Sometimes it can get muddy looking back and trying to erase what has happened, so asking the question from where you'd like to be and working backward is a great way to get the hope you need to execute the plan to get there.

The next question I'd like you to ask yourself is, what are some self-care actions on your list? Every effective plan has action steps to get to the goal. In businesses, they call these KPIs (key performance indicators) that let them know they are heading in the right direction. So what are some indicators that your self-care plan is heading in the right direction? That is what this question will do.

I've included a sample of my self-care action list so you can get an idea of what yours can look like. Feel free to model this or create one that matters most to you. These are just categories that I look through to be present and conscious of how my self-care is developing. In the same way, we want to grow; our self-care mindset should also evolve.

MY SELF-CARE ACTION LIST:

1. **Non-negotiables** - Discipline is a non-negotiable forcing me to be true to myself with the words I speak. This is the practice of holding myself to the highest form of accountability and allowing me to share the skill of reliability and organization with others. Silent Retreats are non-negotiable, allowing me countless opportunities to reflect inwardly and process my thoughts calmly, constructively, and constructively. Good health is a non-negotiable which aligns with the scripture 3 John 1:2, which states, "Dear friend, I pray that you may enjoy good health and that all may go well with you, even as your soul is getting along well." It pleases God when I am in good health. Therefore my goal is to please God with my health.

2. **Important commitments** - A relationship with God is a fundamental commitment to me. This is my source for everything good and would not exist without this commitment. Emotional intelligence is a significant commitment that allows me to understand, use, and manage my own emotions effectively. Gratitude is an important commitment that has become a positive habit that I enjoy daily. Being grateful is foundational to my success in business and my relationship with others. All of these commitments are the YES that I say to myself. We talked about the

stuff we should say "NO" before; these open the door for you to be able to make the "YES" count more.

3. **Hope to accomplish** - Healthy mindset is hoping to achieve that helps me capture every thought and force them to obey God's word within me, rejecting being enslaved to my ideas or the opinions of others. Balance is a hope to accomplish in every area of my life. Balance allows me to adjust quickly to a lifestyle that could be pretty stressful at times. Inner peace is a hope to accomplish minute by minute. The Bible says God gives peace to those He loves. I know God loves me and hope to align with the inner peace that can only come from pleasing Him. Having something you hope to accomplish allows us not to get stuck. There is something we are working towards. These can also be specific milestones you want to reach, that can be running a 5k, getting that degree that you could not get in a previous season in your life. Anything you'd like to accomplish gives you fuel and energy to take care of what's in front of you to get onto the next.

4. **Self-development** - Reading one book weekly is a self-development strategy that gives me access to the knowledge needed for advancement and growth in wisdom, just like Jesus. -Valuing my time is a necessary self-development technique that gives my days, weeks, and months purpose. Each hour has a purpose, and writing them down on paper gives me great pleasure. Saying "YES" to God's will is a self-development practice training my soul to prosper. When my soul prospers, it is because of obedience to God's word and

God's will for my life. This self-development practice has been very profitable for me. Sharing God's goodness and forgiveness with others has been very rewarding.

SELF-CARE CHRONICLES

When I first met Syrenthia almost eight years ago, I knew she was special. Her commitment and passion for parents of children with special needs have been exceptional. As a mom of a special needs young child, I learned how to practice self-care because of her shining example. I've seen her build POCWASN from the ground up. Her mission has always been the same with every event, giveaway, and partnership with parents. She is committed to enabling parents to find their joy despite having children with special needs. The power of community: How I found my voice as a special needs mom

Many challenges come with being a parent of a child with special needs. And when you're in the middle of it all, it can be tough to know what would be helpful for someone else. So I'm sharing how my friend Syrenthia helped me find my voice as a mom of two kids on the autism spectrum.

WHAT IS A SPECIAL NEEDS MOM?

A special needs parent is someone who has raised at least one child with special needs. Our life is different from the average person's because they have the added responsibility of caring for their children and advocating for them. It can be hard to ask for help or reach out, so it's essential to find your voice and not feel ashamed.

The Difficult Journey of Parenting a Special Needs Kid

One of the most complex parts about parenting a special needs child is feeling like you're in this alone. The good news is that there are many resources out there to help. I found my voice when I connected with other parents like Syrenthia, who was in the same boat. We gave each additional support, encouragement, and advice when we needed it most.

How I Found My Voice as a Special Needs Mom Through Syrenthia

I'm a human. I have limitations. And I am a Mom. I'm one of those Moms that you see on Social Media, or maybe in your personal life - the one that's always trying to be perfect. For a long time, I felt like I was never enough for anyone because no matter what I did, someone would find a way to remind me of how much more they could do.

But there was always one person it seemed like no matter what - Syrenthia!

She always encouraged me and helped me out when she could see.

Why We Need Community Support to Heal and Thrive as Special Needs Moms

I know that I am not the only parent who has found her voice through a community. The support of other parents, families, and caregivers gives me the power to speak up for what I need, take care of myself, and make my kids happy.

MY MESSAGE TO ALL PARENTS OF SPECIAL NEEDS CHILDREN

One of the most important things to teach your children with special needs is that there is no such thing as failure. Even if you have a setback or have to take a detour, it's just a lesson that will help them lead a better life in the future. The best way to do this is by letting them take risks and try new things. Accepting their mistakes and helping them learn from them will allow your child to be more independent later on.

ERAINA FERGUSON
Founder of My Good Life

CHAPTER 7

COST OF SELF-CARE

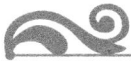

In this book, we've talked about caring for yourself first and the practical strategies and thought patterns that will enable you to do that at the highest level. Even with the ideas shared thus far along with my story, I wanted to make sure the thought of you taking care of yourself would not be missed or be another thing that gets put on the back burner. It's too important for that to happen.

The great screenwriting guru Robert Mckee once said, "Storytelling is the most powerful way to put ideas into the world today." That is why this final chapter of the book includes a series of stories about how others like you have come to learn the value of self-care and its cost.

You've read the self-care chronicles in between the chapters, now hear in more detail the stories of the people who too have been caregivers and their challenges to take care of themselves and the transformation they experienced when they realized caring for themselves first was no longer a cost they could pass up.

You'll not only read their accounts, but I will be providing additional commentary so that you can walk away with the fuel that is needed so you can be sure to drive your self-care journey to the next level. If the commentary sounds like something you've heard in the book already, that is intentional. However, sometimes we need to hear something more than once, sometimes even 100 times, before it sinks in, and the best version is well worth the risk of me sounding like a broken record. So let's dive into these stories, shall we?

ERIN WILSON:

When Syrenthia asked me to write this, I thought, "How can I write about self-care and not feel like a fraud?" My son has severe Autism, and when he was young, my only self-care was making sure I brushed my teeth every day. My respite was going to the grocery store by myself, and my therapist was crying in the car while driving to his appointments. His intervention became everything. I rejoiced in all of his baby steps but felt like a failure when he did not make better progress. Now that he is almost 18, I have gained some perspective. I know that self-care is really how I internally react to life. I also know that I can accept, forgive, and love myself. That is when real sweetness, contentment, and relaxation enter my soul.

Syrenthia's Commentary:
Did you notice the guilt in Erin's story? While she rejoiced in all of her son's baby steps, she still felt like a failure for the time he did not make better progress. This external pressure can bring a caregiver to their knees and have them feel bad about themselves.

So when did the change come from Erin? When she gained perspective! That perspective allowed her to do three things, accept, forgive, and love herself. Remember the chapter on self-forgiveness? The chat about having compassion for yourself and also being patient? These are all the things that Erin's soul needed. The result was sweetness, contentment, and the ability to finally relax. Are you feeling guilty about something right now? Is it tied to disappointing yourself or the expectations of the people around you, or the environments in which you find yourself? It's critical that we are able to pause and spot first what we are feeling and secondly, what is causing the emotions we are feeling. It's only then can we revise our approach to caring for ourselves.

ELLIE:

On this journey, I have realized that self-care is critical when providing for a special needs child because when I don't feel good about myself, I can't be my best self for my child. As a special needs parent I try to balance self-care and my job as a parent by making time each week for my physical health. I have been fortunate to be able to take CrossFit classes and make a commitment to exercising a few days a week. Self-care has been really critical to helping me let go of stress. I have formed connections with others who are committed to their wellness, which has inspired me to continue. I exercise at least 3-4 days a week doing CrossFit and Zumba classes. I have more energy and I feel happier. My overall physical health has improved and I have been motivated to try new things like running my first 5k on my 40th birthday. Self-care through exercise has helped my mental and physical health greatly. In turn, it makes me more capable to tackle the daily challenges that I face as a special needs parent.

Syrenthia's Commentary:
What was the catalyst to Ellie's feeling more capable to tackle the daily challenges she faced as a special needs parent? It was through focusing on her physical self-care. Self-care is a multi-faceted approach. Like our legs are a part of our bodies and work together with the other body parts we have so it is when it comes to our self-care. Ellie's confidence came from putting an emphasis on her physical care. Incorporating CrossFit classes along with Zumba classes not only improved her overall physical health, but there she was able to find community by making connections with others who were committed to their wellness. This is the environment piece that we talked about previously.

Is your environment supportive of the goals you set for yourself? And the part that truly put a smile on my face is seeing Ellie's enthusiasm to try new things, like running her first 5k on her 40th birthday. If that doesn't sound like "I Care For Me First," I don't know what does. Let me ask you this question, what are some new things you have that you want to try? Perhaps you've been putting it off for a while or didn't think you could get to it with everything you already have on your plate. I'd like you to revisit that list or make one now if you haven't done so yet. You do not have to wait for your 40th birthday or a specific milestone to get started on this. You can begin thinking about it and working towards that right now.

ATIAI:

What would be the cost of self-care if you didn't practice it? When asked this question, I first thought about how much money I spend a month. After thinking about it, I realized that this was so much deeper. I am an Applied Behavior Analyst program manager for children with autism. I create behavior intervention plans and supervise the effectiveness of the plans weekly. I work in schools and homes with a caseload of 20. Sometimes my days go from 8 am to 10 pm due to direct sessions and reports. My days can also be from Monday to Saturday, leaving no time to get a massage or socialize. I have high blood pressure because of my lack of self-care, with readings reaching 198/111. My skin has broken out, and I am missing out on moments and events with those I love most. These moments are times that I will never get back. Not practicing self-care has cost me my health, social life, and living the best possible life I could live to become the best version of myself. When we deny ourselves self-care, the ultimate cost becomes our future selves.

Syrenthia's Commentary:
What an opening question Atiai proposed. "What would be the cost of self-care if you didn't practice it?" When it comes to investing in anything, we often think about the benefits of making that investment, but not everyone is driven or motivated by gain. I've heard the opposite. Many people are motivated or driven by the fear of loss. This means you may take action more if you are aware of what you have to lose if you do not act. This is what the question allows Atiai to examine. The question revealed how expensive not practicing self-care is. She shared with us about her physical health, things we can see like high blood pressure and skin breaking out, but I would argue what was more expensive were those moments she spoke of that she would never have back—missing moments and events with those that she loved most. We cannot repurchase past time, so Atiai's account is a great reminder to us all to buy our future with our present choices and decisions.

JAIME:

Fortunately, I have always placed a heavy emphasis on self-care; not to say that I've never had a lapse in implementing it. It's safe for me to say that if I hadn't had those moments of me trying to give 100% when I only had about 40% left in me, I never would have realized just how ineffective I was at completing anything that needed to be done. Everyone's idea of "recharging" is probably a bit different than the next person, but for me, I NEED sleep. It's not about getting my manicures, massages, and mama's night out (although I absolutely enjoy every bit of all of that and I make sure to schedule it in), this mama just has to get her zzzzs in to make her happy, calm, and most of all, functional. Long story short, having a car is great, but if there's no gas in the tank is it going to get you where you need to be?

Syrenthia's Commentary:

Have you tried to give 100% when you had only 40% left in you? We've all been there right? That place where no one else is going to do it and you have to step in and do it, but have we paused to see how effective that effort was? I love the illustration that Jaime shared at the end about having a car is great, but if it has no gas in the tank is it going to get you to where you need to be? No. When it comes to filling up your car with fuel, it can look different for different people. Take time to find what does it for you. I've shared in this book what I do personally to serve as an inspiration not as instructions of what you need to do for you specifically. Like Jaime, maybe sleep is the thing you need more than anything else to be happy, calm, and functional. What do you need to be those three things right now? Is it a massage? A vacation? Discover what your recharge looks like so that you can get where you need to be and be who you are capable of being.

PORTIA:

I used to think that self-care was a secluded club that I obviously was not privy to OR if invited, I wouldn't be able to maintain the membership requirements needed to be apart. After having four boys (one with autism), the word "self" seemed to be null and void. Any and everything pertaining to me, or my needs, were swallowed up in responsibilities. I was ok with that because my children are my heart and their needs are my priority. Sleeping, eating a decent meal, exercising, working on my goals and taking a breather would have to wait, no matter the length of time. My focus was everything." However, there's a price for giving your all. Your children may be cradled in your love and care, but you are often left depleted. Exhausted. Fear and worry grip your soul at the mere thought of walking away to do anything for yourself, even briefly. Decompressing appears impossible, but it brings guilt as if "me" time is frowned upon. It ponders the "what-if" questions and causes you to always think safer than sorry. But last year slapped me with an awakening. I became sick with a virus that made it difficult to walk. It then traveled and struck a chord with my facial muscles, causing Bell Palsy. It took awhile for me to recover. Although I still tried to go over and beyond, I had to depend on others to help me. I had to relinquish some of my day-to-day and trust that my gems would still be alright. I suffered from a thyroid condition this year and was told that stress and fatigue were factors for both conditions. I have to say I still have not completely learned my lesson.

My second born has autism—and the reality of routine requires much. Majority of it comes from the one he has built his livelihood on, me. It's not easy, and I know I'm not the only one trying to balance holding an overwhelming day and night in one hand and a piece of yourself needing to smell the roses sometimes in the other. Self-care means taking the initiative to practice safeguarding or enhancing your total well-being. It takes time to respect yourself spiritually, physically, emotionally, and mentally. I still struggle, but I'm trying to recognize my limits better. I'm making an effort to pay attention to myself and not just to the precious ones around my heart. I realize that care for me has been deleted from my norm. I have to figure out how to change my environment to not only cater to my gems but also embrace my desires and essentials. How can I feed myself without feeling like the world surrounding me is judging me? I'm a work in progress. I go to the grocery store daily and will, at times, watch a Hallmark movie that I taped weeks prior. That's part of my self-care routine. I have a long way to go, but I'm at a turtle's pace. I've come to understand that if I do not take some time for myself, even if it's a few minutes each day, I won't be any good for the ones who need me—the ones I love. It's a step I have to take.

Syrenthia's Commentary:
Portia's story is all too familiar. Embedded in the story are shame and guilt, forever thinking that "me" could be a thing again. We can see that weight can be too much to bear and open up Pandora's box to many other problems. Too often, our depth overlooking our self-care can make us feel defeated even in starting.

From Portia's story, the takeaway is that the slow turtle pace is a lot faster than no pace. Do not worry about having a perfect self-care routine. Too many things are not in our control as caregivers, and as she shared, habits have often been built almost like you are the sun of someone else's world. With that reality, practice grace and patience. As they say, Rome was not built in a day; every step you take is one step closer to showing up as your best self and giving you what you need. Do not despise small beginnings. So many things that are giants started off tiny. Give yourself what you need, even if it's a bit at a time.

I hope you realize that you are not alone in your journey towards caring for yourself first. It's a fight that is not easy, nor is it one that will happen overnight. I'm interested in hearing what your account is; what is your story? Sometimes, in sharing your story, you can uncover the power you need to help write a better next chapter of your life. At the end of this book, you'll see how you can reach out to me so I can give you the invitation to be "ME" again.

CONCLUSION

So what's next?

This entire book was a cry of the heart. Whose heart? Yours. Your heart is screaming for the love and care you share to go outwards and go inwards. For the love and care to not be sent your way last but for it to be sent first to you so that you could be in a position to give the best form of love and care out without costing you your sanity and putting the lives of those you are called to care for at risk.

If this were commonplace or so easy, this book would have no place, and I would have no reason to write it. Therefore, this book's strategies, tips, and charges will get used. Do not let that discourage you or stop you from pursuing what the title of this book asks you to care for yourself first.

Through the stories of the many ladies in this book who shared not knowing what self-care was, to feeling an overwhelming feeling of shame and guilt as they tend to their own needs, you can see firsthand that self-care is no longer an activity of luxury. Instead, it's one of necessity.

It took me years of barely any sleep and living as a parent raising autism and failing to put myself first to grasp the courage to care for myself. However, the importance of practicing self-care ultimately saved my life, and it's why I will continue to champion the message of self-care for caregivers through both the Parents of Children with All Special Needs (POCWASN) and the self-care services provided through iCare4MeFirst.

On your next journey, let me know how you're putting yourself first, how you are caring for yourself first, and do not forget to share your photos and your stories with me so that I may share with the community of caregivers in the world. You matter, and let no one or anything tell you any different.

ACKNOWLEDGMENTS

Exodus 15:26, For I am the Lord who heals you.

Writing a book was more complicated than I thought, but it is way more rewarding than I could ever imagine. But, of course, none of this would be possible without my Heavenly Father, who was with me through my greatest battle and provided Mary (Granny) as a vessel and support system while raising Autism.

To the late Stephen Moore, may you rest well. Thank you for teaching me the importance of practicing emotional self-care and providing me with strategies for self-preservation. I am forever grateful to you.

To Yvonne Brooks, Thank you for showing me the right path, to live a simple life, and always finding what is important to ME. It would be impossible to list all you have done to encourage me throughout the years of being a vessel. I'm filled with gratitude for the love and continuous support.

To Mohamed AlRafi, I admire and appreciate your leadership; you are a Blessing to Caregivers. Thank you for the support and time you have invested in all projects in the Special Needs Community.

To Sean Mead, You are indeed a gift from God. Thank you for being such a vital part of my life.

I am filled with gratitude from your support to the providers who invested their time in assisting me with my daily self-care needs.

To my company and two co-workers who supported me through an unveiling time, without the experience, this book would not exist.

To my Granny, may you continue resting in heaven. I'm beyond blessed for the long talk and eternally grateful that you taught me how to parent a child with a disability from a distance. I love you forever!

Thank you for your unconditional love and support and for walking hand in hand on this life journey with me to my amazing husband, Bill.

To my kids: Stephen, Amber, Bill D., and Victoria, I love you dearly. Life is not about finding yourself; it's about creating yourself.

INSPIRATIONAL QUOTES TO LIVE BY:

"I listen to God's voice in everything I do and everywhere I go. He's the one that will keep me on track."

"If you never learn how to deal with problems you'll never reach your potential. The closer I come to my purpose the more I come in contact with problems. The problem is not the problem, it was always my perception of it. I learned that purpose and problems go together. The whole point of problems is to pull you out of purpose. God is using my life to prove a point to people."

"Love yourself enough to set boundaries. Your time and energy are precious. You get to choose how you use it. You teach people how to treat you by deciding what you will and won't accept."
—Anna Taylor

"Fear does not stop death. It stops life. And worrying does not take away from tomorrow's troubles. It takes away today's peace."

"Without rain nothing grows. Learn to embrace the storms in your life."

"I am my own rescue. I like myself today, and you are 'like' for me is just extra."

"The heaviest burdens we carry are the thoughts in our head."

"You have been criticizing yourself for years and it hasn't worked. Try approving yourself and see what happens."
—Louis Hay

"No person alive can build you up without learning the pieces."

"As humans, we aren't only affected by what happens to us but by the filter through which we view what happens to us."

"The secret to failure is trying to please everybody."

"Your value does not depend on what other people think about you. Value development is a job done in silence. So give yourself the gift of silence to care for your inner being."

"Gratitude is the most valuable experience in life."

"Gratitude makes sense of our past, brings peace for today, and creates a vision for tomorrow."
—Melody Beattie

"In all codependent relationships, the rescuer needs the victim as much as the victim needs the rescuer."
—Barbara De Angelis

"These are the happiest moments of your life; when the real you comes out. When you don't care about the past, you don't worry about the future. You are childlike."
—Miguel Angel Ruiz

"One can choose to go back toward safety or forward toward growth. Growth must be chosen again and again, and fear must be overcome again and again."
—Abraham Maslow

"Always forward, never backward!"
—Syrenthia

"Just when you feel you have no time to relax, know that this is the moment you most need to make time to relax."
—Matt Haiq

"We need quiet time to examine our lives openly and honestly. Spending quiet time alone gives your mind an opportunity to renew itself and create order."
—Susan Taylor

"Solitude is when I place my chaos to rest and awaken my inner peace."
—Nikki Rowe

ABOUT THE AUTHOR

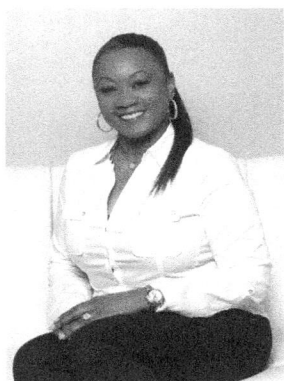

Syrenthia Colino is the founder and CEO of iCare4MeFirst and POCWASN which is a non-profit organization that provides services and resources to caregivers in need of self-care.

At the age of 19, her 2-year-old son Stephen was diagnosed with autism. She became a strong advocate thereafter navigating the endless maze of doctors, clinics, and treatment centers.

While being the primary caregiver for her son for 20 years, she reached a breaking point where she became emotionally exhausted and enlisted the support of close friends and family to rejuvenate and jump-start her life.

Her process was an endless and deliberate amount of self-care that gave birth to the organizations she heads, now helping other caregivers put their self-care at the forefront. When not caring for herself, you can find her speaking and coaching other caregivers on how to prioritize their self-care so they can be good for themselves and those they love. She currently resides in Southern California.

Ways to Connect With Syrenthia

Instagram:
@POCWASN
@Syrenthia_Colino

Blogs:
iCare4MeFirst.com
SelfCare4Caregivers.org

Facebook:
www.Facebook.com/POCWASN

Website:
www.POCWASN.org

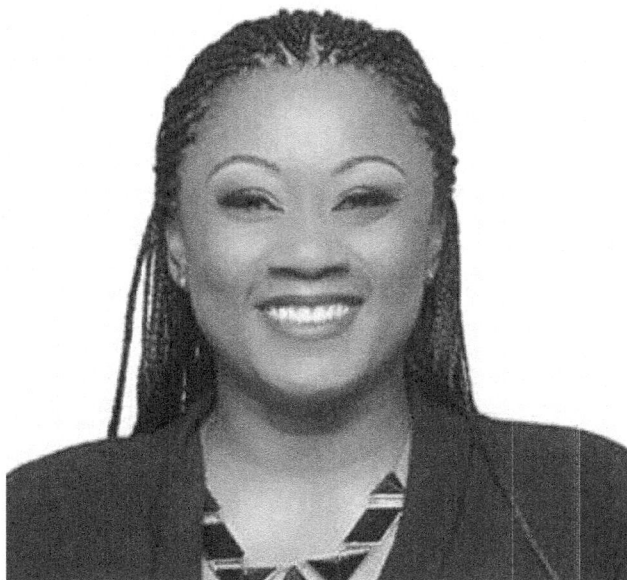

Did you know Syrenthia and her team offer speaking engagements geared towards caregivers?

If you have an event that needs a speaker who understands the rigors of being a caregiver and wants to promote self-care to them, look no further than Syrenthia Colino and her team of speakers. You may reach her at www.iCare4MeFirst.com.

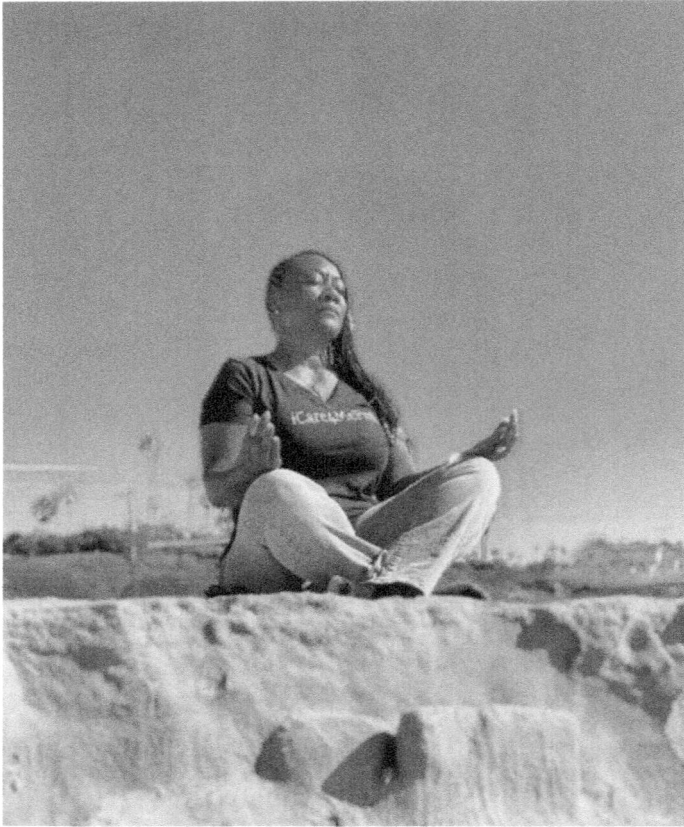

ARE YOU A CAREGIVER WHO COULD USE SOME GUIDANCE ON DEVELOPING YOUR OWN SELF-CARE ROUTINE?

Syrenthia provides coaching for caregivers of all kinds who need to put their care first. To schedule a coaching session, send an email to syrenthiacolinio@gmail. com with the subject line: "Coaching Needed"

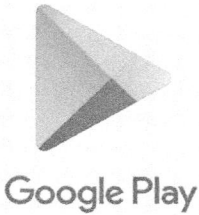

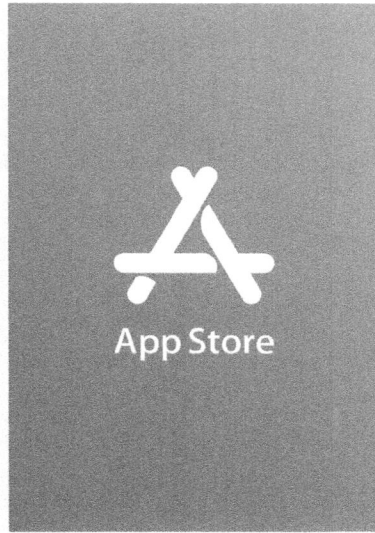

Our app is live on the Google Play Store, where you can download it today! Simply type in the search bar, "iCare4MeFirst", the download. In the app, you will find additional resources that you can use to help with your self-care journey, including blog posts, articles, and lots more. The iOS/Apple version is coming soon!

Made in the USA
Las Vegas, NV
26 November 2022

60373932R00062